I0774820

HOLISTIC APPROACHES TO HOLISTIC DENTISTRY AND ORAL HEALTH

Expert Guide to natural remedies, mindful practices, and integrative strategies for achieving Optimal Health

DR. CHRIS FRIEDRICH

Copyright © 2023 by Chris Friedrich

All rights reserved.

Disclaimer

This book on Herbal Remedies is intended solely for informational and educational purposes.

The content provided within this book is based on general knowledge and should not be considered as professional advice. The author is not a licensed medical professional, and the information presented here is not intended to diagnose, treat, cure, or prevent any disease.

Readers are advised to consult with qualified healthcare professionals before initiating any herbal remedies or making changes to their existing health regimen. The author and publisher disclaim any responsibility for any adverse effects or consequences resulting from the use of information contained in this book.

It's important to note that the content of this book is not endorsed by any specific platform or affiliated with any product or service.

The author does not receive any compensation or benefits from the promotion of specific herbal products or brands.

Readers should exercise their discretion and judgment when applying the information from this book, and they are encouraged to conduct further research and seek guidance from healthcare professionals to make informed decisions about their health and well-being.

In-depth and perceptive, "Holistic Approaches to Holistic Dentistry and Oral Health" explores the complex field of holistic dentistry, offering a thorough examination of its tenets, applications, and importance in modern oral healthcare. The introduction provides a basic understanding of holistic dentistry, clarifying its definition and highlighting its vital role in promoting overall well-being. The main goal of the book is to offer a holistic viewpoint, integrating oral health with more general aspects of the mind and body.

The first chapter, "The Foundations of Holistic Dentistry," takes the reader on a historical tour, explaining the philosophy and basic ideas of holistic dentistry as well as how it developed. The story then moves on to the integration of oral health, body, and mind, providing a holistic framework that goes beyond conventional dental techniques.

In the following chapters, different facets of holistic dentistry are presented, with particular attention to oral hygiene, nutritional factors, and biological dentistry. Chapter 2, "Biological Dentistry," examines the significance of mercury-free dentistry, safe amalgam filling removal, and the use of materials that are compatible with biology. Chapter 3 delves into the critical role that nutrition plays in holistic dentistry, outlining appropriate foods and nutritional supplements for the best possible oral health.

A thorough guide to maintaining a balanced and harmonious oral care routine is provided in Chapters 4 and 5, which discuss holistic oral hygiene practices and the mind-body connection in dentistry, respectively. These sections cover everything from natural and non-toxic toothpaste to stress management techniques that impact oral health.

In addition, the book delves into integrative therapies, pediatric dentistry, and environmental sustainability in the field of dentistry.

Chapter 6 provides an overview of holistic dental care by examining the use of acupuncture, homeopathy, and herbal medicine.

Chapter 7 emphasizes the importance of early holistic oral care and preventive measures for children.

Chapter 8 extends the holistic paradigm to environmental concerns by talking about eco-friendly dental practices and green dentistry.

"Holistic Approaches to Holistic Dentistry and Oral Health" is a valuable resource for dental professionals, researchers, and anyone seeking a thorough understanding of the integration of holistic principles with dental practices.

Chapters 9 and 10 discuss specific dental issues and the future landscape of holistic dentistry.

From natural remedies for cavities to holistic solutions for tooth sensitivity, the book offers practical insights.

The final chapter anticipates the future of holistic dentistry, discussing emerging trends, research, and innovation, thereby encapsulating the book's forward-thinking approach.

Overview

In contrast to conventional dentistry, which frequently focuses only on treating dental problems, holistic dentistry seeks to prevent problems and optimize health through a patient-centered approach. Holistic dentistry is a comprehensive approach to oral health care that goes beyond the traditional focus on treating symptoms and emphasizes the interconnectedness of oral health with overall well-being.

Holistic dentistry considers the whole person, taking into account physical, emotional, and spiritual aspects.

What Holistic Dentistry Is Defined As

Holistic dentists consider the impact of dental treatments on the overall well-being of their patients.

They use biocompatible materials, focus on preventive measures, and emphasize patient education to empower individuals in managing their oral health. Holistic dentistry, also known as biological or integrative dentistry, is based on the belief that oral health is inseparable from the health of the entire body. This approach recognizes that the mouth is a gateway to the body and that problems in the oral cavity can impact systemic health.

The Value Of Holistic Strategies For Dental Health

A more comprehensive and long-lasting approach to oral health care is promoted by holistic approaches, which recognize the significant influence oral health can have on a person's overall well-being. Traditional dentistry, on the other hand, frequently treats symptoms in isolation, ignoring the possible systemic effects of dental procedures and materials. Holistic dentistry, on the other hand, acknowledges the dynamic relationship between oral health and systemic health; for instance, gum disease has been linked to several systemic conditions, including diabetes and cardiovascular disease.

Furthermore, the use of biocompatible materials is critical to holistic dentistry. While traditional dental materials, like mercury amalgam fillings, may present health risks to patients, holistic dentists place a higher priority on using materials that are in harmony with the body, reducing the possibility of negative reactions and long-term health problems. This approach is consistent with the larger trend in healthcare toward customized and patient-centered care that takes individual sensitivities and preferences into account.

Synopsis Of The Work

Using a thorough analysis of case studies and research findings, the book on holistic approaches to holistic dentistry and oral health aims to provide a comprehensive exploration of this evolving field. It also explores the integration of holistic dentistry with conventional approaches, fostering a more inclusive and collaborative model of oral health care. Finally, the book delves into the fundamental principles of holistic dentistry, examining its historical roots and philosophical foundations.

In keeping with the tenets of holistic dentistry, which emphasize a partnership between the dentist and the patient, the book also emphasizes the importance of patient education. By encouraging a more thorough comprehension of the relationships between oral and systemic health, the book hopes to stimulate a proactive approach to preventive care.

To sum up, this book is an invaluable tool for dental professionals, students, and anyone else who wants to learn about and embrace holistic approaches to oral health. It bridges the theory-practice divide and provides insights into holistic dentistry's transformative potential in promoting overall well-being. As the field develops, this book adds to the ongoing discussion about how to incorporate holistic principles into mainstream dental care, thereby reshaping oral health for a more integrated and patient-centered approach.

CHAPTER 1
THE BASIS OF HOLISTIC DENTISTRY

Dentistry has evolved from a reductionist model to one that acknowledges the complex interplay between various factors influencing oral health. The historical evolution of holistic dentistry is characterized by a departure from conventional practices and an embrace of a more patient-centered, integrative philosophy.

Holistic dentistry represents a paradigm shift in the approach to oral health care, extending beyond the traditional focus on symptoms and treatment of dental issues to encompass a comprehensive understanding of the interconnectedness between oral health, overall health, and the well-being of an individual.

The Development Of Holistic Dentistry Throughout History

The origins of holistic dentistry can be found in the mid-1900s when pioneers in the field started questioning accepted dental practices.

Early proponents, like Dr. Weston A. Price, highlighted the symbiotic relationship between diet and oral health and the impact of nutrition on dental health.

This was a departure from the predominant focus on invasive treatments and sparked a broader understanding of preventive measures and lifestyle factors influencing oral health. Over time, holistic dentistry has changed in response to new scientific findings, societal changes, and an increasing understanding of the connection between oral health and systemic health.

The Foundations And Ideology Of Holistic Dentistry

Holistic dentists emphasize the use of biocompatible materials in dental treatments, acknowledging the potential impact of dental materials on the body and overall health. Additionally, the philosophy of holistic dentistry incorporates a patient-centered approach, viewing individuals as unique entities with diverse needs that extend beyond mere dental procedures.

These principles and unique approaches set holistic dentistry apart from conventional dental practices. One core principle is the recognition of the mouth as a gateway to overall health. Holistic dentists also understand that oral health issues can have far-reaching effects on systemic well-being.

Combining Physical, Mental, And Dental Health

The integration of mind, body, and oral health is the cornerstone of holistic dentistry.

It acknowledges the profound relationship between individual well-being and oral health, as well as the role that psychological and emotional factors play in oral health outcomes, including temporomandibular joint disorders and bruxism. Holistic dentists frequently work in conjunction with other healthcare professionals, such as psychologists, nutritionists, and holistic health practitioners, to address the wider range of factors that impact patient well-being.

This multidisciplinary approach guarantees a more thorough and integrated care model that takes into account the complex interplay between mental, physical, and oral health.

holistic dentistry's roots are in a historical development that questions conventional dental practices, embracing a philosophy and set of principles that emphasize the connection between oral health and overall well-being.

Holistic dentistry is distinguished by the integration of mind, body, and oral health, which directs practitioners toward a patient-centered approach that takes into account the various factors influencing an individual's health.

As the field develops further, holistic dentistry serves as a testament to the significance of taking an all-encompassing and integrative approach to oral healthcare.

CHAPTER 2
DENTAL BIOLOGY

To provide comprehensive and individualized care, Biological Dentistry emphasizes a holistic approach to oral health, taking into account the interconnectedness of the mouth with the body's overall well-being. This approach acknowledges the impact of dental procedures and materials on systemic health and advocates for practices that promote harmony within the body. Practitioners who understand Biological Dentistry delve into the complex relationship between oral and systemic health, acknowledging the influence of oral conditions on various bodily functions.

Mercury-Free Dentistry advocates prioritize the use of alternative materials for dental fillings, avoiding the potential hazards associated with mercury exposure. This approach is in line with the principles of Biological Dentistry by protecting patients from potential systemic health issues related to mercury toxicity. Dental amalgam, which has been widely used for decades in fillings, has raised concerns due to its mercury content. Mercury is a toxic substance that can potentially pose health risks.

Biological Dentistry places a high priority on safety protocols to minimize potential health risks for patients and dental professionals. One of the most important components of its protocols is the safe removal of amalgam fillings. Practitioners in this field follow strict guidelines to ensure safe removal procedures, which include using protective measures like rubber dams, high-volume suction, and specialized ventilation systems to minimize the inhalation and absorption of mercury vapors during the removal process.

Biological Dentistry emphasizes the selection of dental materials that promote overall health and well-being, avoiding substances that may have negative systemic effects. This approach involves thorough patient assessment to identify any potential sensitivities or allergies, allowing for the customization of treatment plans using materials that are in harmony with the patient's unique biological makeup. Biological Materials in Dentistry represent a shift toward the use of biocompatible materials that are harmonious with the body's natural systems. This includes materials that are less likely to elicit adverse reactions or sensitivities.

Encouraging Mercury-Free Dentistry, Safe Removal of Amalgam Fillings, and the use of Biological Materials in Dentistry, among other initiatives, practitioners hope to provide holistic dental care that prioritizes both oral and systemic health. This paradigm shift in dentistry reflects a commitment to patient safety, personalized treatment, and a broader understanding of the impact of dental practices on the body as a whole. In summary, Biological Dentistry is a comprehensive and patient-centric approach that recognizes the intricate relationship between oral health and overall well-being.

CHAPTER 3
NUTRITIONAL ASPECTS OF ORAL HEALTH

In the field of holistic dentistry, which goes beyond traditional dental procedures to adopt a more all-encompassing approach to oral health, nutritional factors are crucial. This holistic viewpoint recognizes the interdependence of different body systems and the impact of nutrition on maintaining healthy teeth and gums.

Holistic dentists stress the importance of nutrition as a cornerstone in maintaining overall oral health.

A core idea in holistic dentistry is the role that nutrition plays in maintaining oral health. According to this view, eating a diet rich in nutrients and balanced helps prevent dental problems. Vital nutrients, like vitamins and minerals, are important for keeping teeth and gums healthy. For example, vitamin D is known to be important for calcium absorption, which is vital for dental health, and vitamin C is known to help form collagen, which is necessary for gum tissue integrity. Patients who practice holistic dentistry are encouraged to follow a diet that includes these vital nutrients to optimize their body's innate ability to handle oral health issues.

Another essential component of holistic dentistry is foods for healthy teeth and gums. Here, the focus is on selecting foods that support oral health rather than just avoiding those that may cause dental issues. Eating a diet high in fruits and vegetables, especially those high in fiber helps produce saliva and keeps the mouth's pH levels at an ideal level. Foods that are high in calcium and phosphorus also aid in the remineralization of tooth enamel. Holistic dentistry helps people make educated food decisions by including a range of nutrient-dense options that have a positive effect on oral health.

As a crucial part of holistic dentistry, nutritional supplements act as a supplement to dietary practices. This is because holistic dentistry understands that modern lifestyles may not always allow for optimal nutritional intake through food alone, and it advocates for specific supplements to address specific oral health needs.

For instance, omega-3 fatty acids have been linked to anti-inflammatory effects, which may benefit people with periodontal issues. It may also recommend calcium and vitamin D supplements for people whose deficiencies affect their dental health. Holistic dentistry acknowledges the importance of obtaining nutrients from whole foods, but it also recognizes the role that supplements play in filling nutritional gaps and promoting overall oral health.

holistic dentistry emphasizes the vital role that nutrition plays in promoting optimal oral health. It goes beyond conventional dental practices by recognizing the interdependence of body systems and the influence that nutrition has on overall health. By comprehending the role that nutrition plays in holistic dentistry, people can make educated decisions about their diet and lifestyle, which can help prevent dental problems and promote overall health and well-being. By emphasizing foods that are good for teeth and gums and using nutritional supplements sparingly, holistic dentistry offers a sophisticated oral care strategy that incorporates dietary practices into the larger context of overall health and well-being.

CHAPTER 4
HOLISTIC ORAL HYGIENE PRACTICES

The use of natural and non-toxic toothpaste is a cornerstone of holistic oral hygiene practices, which emphasize a comprehensive approach to oral health that takes into account the interconnectedness of the mouth and the rest of the body. This approach goes beyond conventional dentistry by recognizing the impact of oral health on overall well-being.

Non-Toxic And Natural Toothpaste

Using toothpaste free of dangerous chemicals and additives that are often present in conventional dental products is recommended by holistic dentistry. Fluoride, sodium lauryl sulfate, and artificial sweeteners are just a few of the ingredients that are commonly found in traditional toothpaste and have been linked to several health issues. Natural toothpaste substitutes, on the other hand, usually contain ingredients like baking soda, essential oils, and herbal extracts.

These ingredients not only support oral health but also enhance overall wellness. The holistic approach emphasizes the value of promoting health without compromising other areas of the body.

Oil Pulling's Advantages

Oil pulling is an age-old holistic practice that entails swishing oil—typically coconut or sesame oil—in the mouth for a predetermined amount of time. Oil-pulling proponents assert that this method helps eliminate toxins, bacteria, and plaque from the oral cavity, promoting better oral health and possibly impacting overall wellness. The procedure is thought to enhance oral hygiene by preventing cavities, reducing bad breath, and improving gum health.

Studies have suggested that oil pulling may have a positive impact on oral hygiene; however, there is a lack of scientific evidence to support these claims. The holistic perspective on oil pulling highlights the connection between oral health and wider health outcomes, strengthening the significance of considering the whole person.

Scraping The Tongue And Detoxifying The Mouth

Using a tongue scraper (usually made of plastic or metal), one can remove bacteria and toxins from the surface of the tongue by gently cleaning its coating. Based on holistic dentistry principles, tongue scraping helps the body's natural detoxification processes by preventing the reabsorption of toxins into the bloodstream.

It also enhances taste perception, freshens breath, and promotes overall oral health. Although there is limited scientific evidence supporting the detoxification aspect of tongue scraping, it is widely acknowledged as a low-risk, easy-to-use technique that supports the holistic approach to oral health.

Natural Dental Treatments Using Herbs

Herbal approaches are used in holistic dentistry to acknowledge the potential benefits of plant-based remedies. Some herbs, like calendula, neem, and aloe vera, have been used for their antimicrobial, anti-inflammatory, and healing properties; neem, for example, is known to fight bacteria, reduce plaque, and support gum health; aloe vera's calming qualities can help heal and reduce inflammation in the oral cavity; calendula is another herb used in holistic dentistry.

Herbal approaches are aligned with the holistic philosophy by emphasizing the use of natural, plant-derived substances to enhance oral health without the possible side effects associated with

The use of natural and non-toxic toothpaste, oil pulling, tongue scraping, and herbal approaches reflect the holistic philosophy of promoting health while minimizing potential harm. These practices emphasize the importance of viewing oral health as an integral part of the whole body, emphasizing the need for personalized and comprehensive care. While scientific evidence may vary in supporting these holistic concepts, their integration into oral care routines aligns with a growing interest in natural and holistic approaches to health and wellness. In conclusion, holistic oral hygiene practices encompass a range of approaches that extend beyond traditional dentistry to consider the interconnectedness of oral health with overall well-being.

CHAPTER 5
DENTISTRY'S MIND-BODY CONNECTION

The concept of the mind-body connection in dentistry signifies a paradigm shift in the field's understanding of oral health, recognizing the complex relationship between mental health and dental outcomes. Stress, anxiety, and psychological factors are significant factors that contribute to the emergence and development of various oral health issues.

Dental professionals are beginning to understand the importance of treating patients holistically, taking into account both their physical and mental states. This shift in perspective is a departure from traditional methods that only address the physical aspects of oral care.

Stress's Impact On Dental Health

Stress is a commonplace aspect of contemporary life and has been found to have a significant impact on oral health.

Long-term stress can lead to the development and aggravation of several dental conditions, from temporomandibular joint disorders to periodontal diseases. The biological mechanisms that link stress and oral health are complex and include immune system modulation, hormonal imbalances, and altered oral hygiene behaviors. The release of stress hormones, such as cortisol, may compromise the body's defenses against oral pathogens, increasing the risk of infection. Additionally, stress-induced behaviors, such as teeth grinding (bruxism), can cause enamel erosion and jaw pain. Holistic dentistry, in addressing stress and its impact on oral health.

Techniques For Relaxation And Mindfulness

To promote holistic oral health, mindfulness, and relaxation techniques have become essential tools. The physiological effects of stress on the oral cavity can be greatly reduced by incorporating practices like deep breathing, progressive muscle relaxation, and mindfulness, which have their roots in ancient contemplative traditions. Mindfulness, when applied to dentistry, can empower patients to approach dental procedures with a calmer mindset, reducing anxiety and potentially alleviating conditions exacerbated by stress. Dental professionals are increasingly integrating mindfulness-based interventions into their practices, realizing the potential benefits .

Integrated Methods For Handling Dental Fear

Dental anxiety remains a pervasive challenge for both patients and practitioners, often leading to avoidance of necessary dental care.

 Holistic approaches to managing dental anxiety encompass a spectrum of interventions that address the root causes of fear and discomfort. Beyond traditional sedation techniques, holistic dentistry explores alternative methods such as aromatherapy, music therapy, and biofeedback. Aromatherapy, using essential oils with calming properties, aims to create a soothing environment in the dental office. Similarly, music therapy harnesses the therapeutic effects of music to alleviate anxiety and enhance relaxation during dental procedures. Biofeedback techniques enable patients to gain awareness and control over physiological responses, allowing them to actively participate in managing their anxiety.

These holistic strategies not only target the symptoms but also consider the emotional and psychological aspects of dental anxiety, fostering a patient-centered approach to oral healthcare.

CHAPTER 6
INTEGRATIVE ORAL HEALTH THERAPIES

Because dental health is so important to overall health, holistic dentistry emphasizes the integration of different therapeutic modalities to provide comprehensive care. This kind of dentistry acknowledges the connection between an individual's overall health and oral health, recognizing that problems in the oral cavity can affect systemic health and vice versa. Of the many integrative therapies that are available, acupuncture, homeopathy, and herbal medicine have drawn attention for their potential benefits to oral wellness.

Dental Acupuncture: An Overview

The ancient Chinese medical practice of acupuncture involves inserting thin needles into specific body points to facilitate energy flow and healing. In the context of dentistry, acupuncture has become recognized as a complementary therapy with potential benefits for a range of oral health issues. Studies have shown that acupuncture may be useful in treating dental anxiety, minimizing pain during dental procedures, and even relieving temporomandibular joint (TMJ) disorders.

The stimulation of specific acupuncture points is thought to affect the nervous system, modify pain perception, and improve the body's inherent healing abilities. Although more research is required to confirm the effectiveness of acupuncture in treating particular dental conditions, its holistic approach is consistent with dentistry.

Oral Health And Homeopathy

Homeopathy is an alternative medicine system that dates back to the late 18th century.

Its foundations lie on the ideas of "like cures like" and customized care. For oral health, homeopathic remedies are used to treat a variety of conditions, such as toothaches, gum disease, and oral infections. These remedies are made from natural substances and are thought to stimulate the body's vital force to restore balance and promote healing. Homeopathic practitioners take into account each patient's unique set of symptoms when prescribing remedies, emphasizing a customized approach to oral care. Although there is little scientific evidence to support the effectiveness of homeopathy in dentistry, some patients report positive results, and supporters contend that the system's holistic philosophy aligns with modern dentistry.

Oral Health And Herbal Medicine

Herbal medicine has been employed for centuries across cultures to address various health concerns, and its application in oral wellness is no exception. The use of medicinal plants and herbs in dentistry aligns with the holistic philosophy of addressing oral health within the broader context of overall well-being. Commonly used herbs in oral care include aloe vera, chamomile, and tea tree oil, each recognized for its antimicrobial, anti-inflammatory, and soothing properties.

These natural substances may be incorporated into toothpaste, and mouthwash, or applied topically to address issues such as gum inflammation, oral infections, and bad breath. While herbal medicine holds promise in promoting oral wellness, it is important to note that scientific research on the efficacy and safety of specific herbal remedies in dentistry is an evolving field. Integrative dentistry encourages a cautious and evidence-based approach to the incorporation of herbal medicine into treatment plans, considering both traditional knowledge and contemporary scientific findings.

the integration of integrative therapies like homeopathy, herbal medicine, and acupuncture into dentistry represents a larger movement toward holistic approaches to oral health. These therapies, which have their roots in traditional healing practices, offer distinctive viewpoints and potential advantages that are consistent with integrative dentistry's comprehensive care philosophy. Although more research is required to determine the safety and effectiveness of these approaches in particular dental conditions, their consideration in the context of a customized and patient-centered approach is an example of how dentistry is evolving toward a more holistic and integrated model of healthcare.

CHAPTER 7
HOLISTIC PEDIATRIC DENTISTRY

Recognizing the connection between overall well-being and dental health, holistic pediatric dentistry emphasizes an all-encompassing and integrative approach to treating children's oral health issues. This approach includes a range of concepts intended to promote not only healthy teeth and gums but also a child's overall physical and emotional well-being.

A key tenet of holistic pediatric dentistry is "starting holistic oral care early," which emphasizes the importance of education and early intervention in helping children develop lifelong healthy oral hygiene habits. It also calls for regular dental check-ups for young children and the education of parents about the value of oral hygiene. Pediatric dentists who follow this paradigm may concentrate on making children feel at ease and comfortable during dental visits, as well as lowering anxiety and encouraging a positive association with dental care.

Another essential component of Holistic Pediatric Dentistry is Nutritional Guidelines for Children. Since diet has a direct effect on oral health, holistic dentists promote a healthy, balanced diet that supports overall health as well as optimal dental health. This involves teaching parents about the role that nutrition plays in preventing common childhood dental problems like cavities and gum disease. Particular emphasis is placed on minimizing the consumption of sugary snacks and beverages, increasing the intake of necessary nutrients, and encouraging adequate hydration.

The goal of holistic dentistry is to create a foundation of oral health that goes beyond the mere absence of disease and encompasses overall well-being. One of the main components of the holistic approach is the prevention of oral health issues in children. To this end, proactive measures are stressed, such as regular dental check-ups, the application of dental sealants, and the promotion of good oral hygiene practices. Holistic dentists may also investigate alternative and complementary approaches, like herbal remedies or holistic fluoride alternatives, to enhance preventive care.

Beyond the pediatric realm, holistic approaches to holistic dentistry encompass a more comprehensive outlook on oral health that unites the mind, body, and spirit. These approaches are based on the notion that an individual's overall health is linked to their oral health, emphasizing preventive care, natural remedies, and a patient-centered approach to dentistry.

Addressing the Mind-Body Connection in Holistic Dentistry: Holistic dentistry recognizes the complex interrelationship between mental and physical health and stresses that stress, anxiety, and other emotional factors can have a significant impact on oral health. Its goal is to create a dental environment that takes patients' psychological well-being into account.

To this end, it employs techniques like mindfulness exercises, relaxation exercises, and communication strategies to reduce dental anxiety and foster a positive overall experience.

A key concept in holistic dentistry is biocompatibility in dental materials. Conventional dental materials, like mercury-containing amalgam fillings, have sparked concerns about their possible effects on general health. Holistic dentists place a high priority on using biocompatible materials that are safe for the body and reduce the possibility of negative reactions. Examples of these materials include composite fillings, ceramic restorations, and other materials that are more in line with the body's natural composition.

One of the main principles of holistic approaches is the Impact of Systemic Health on Oral Health; the health of the mouth is thought to be a reflection of the health of the body as a whole, and vice versa. Holistic dentists work in conjunction with other medical professionals to take into account systemic conditions, like diabetes or cardiovascular disease, that may have an impact on oral health. This integrated approach guarantees that dental care is customized to the patient's overall health status, fostering a holistic understanding of well-being.

Combining traditional periodontal therapies like scaling and root planing with holistic interventions like nutritional counseling, herbal remedies, and lifestyle modifications, holistic periodontal care goes beyond conventional treatments for gum disease by addressing the underlying factors causing periodontal issues. Holistic dentistry aims to prevent recurrence and promote long-term oral health by addressing the root causes of periodontal disease.

The term "oral-systemic connection" refers to the interaction between systemic and oral health. Holistic dentists understand that diseases like periodontal disease can have an impact on other medical conditions, diabetes, and cardiovascular health.

By recognizing and treating the oral-systemic connection, they work toward holistic health outcomes that go beyond simply treating oral health.

Holistic dentists prioritize a patient-centered approach, involving individuals in their care and treatment decisions. This concept acknowledges the significance of informed consent and patient education, empowering individuals to actively participate in their oral health journey.

By taking the time to educate patients about treatment options, potential risks, and preventive measures, holistic dentists foster a collaborative and transparent relationship between the patient and the dentist. A fundamental component of holistic dental care is patient-centered and informed decision-making.

Ultimately, holistic dentistry—whether it be in the context of pediatric oral health or a more generalized understanding of oral health—represents a paradigm shift toward a more all-encompassing and patient-centered approach. Through the incorporation of ideas like early intervention, dietary guidelines, preventive measures, addressing the mind-body connection, biocompatibility in dental materials, considering systemic health, holistic periodontal care, comprehending the oral-systemic connection, and encouraging patient-centered decision-making, holistic dentistry aims to raise the bar for dental care by recognizing the interconnectedness of oral health and treating oral conditions.

CHAPTER 8
SUSTAINABLE DENTISTRY AND THE ENVIRONMENT

A paradigm shift in the dental industry, eco-friendly dental practices emphasize the need to minimize the environmental footprint associated with oral healthcare. These practices extend beyond the clinic walls and involve considerations ranging from waste management to the materials used in dental procedures. While dentistry has traditionally focused on oral health, it is now increasingly recognizing its impact on the environment, which has led to the emergence of sustainable practices within the field.

Environmental Responsibility And Green Dental Practices

As a branch of sustainable dentistry, green dentistry is a broad approach that incorporates ecologically conscious principles into all aspects of dental care. It highlights the use of eco-friendly materials, energy-efficient technologies, and waste-reduction strategies. Green dentistry also extends beyond the clinical setting to administrative practices like the use of energy-efficient appliances and lighting, as well as administrative procedures like electronic record-keeping to minimize paper use. The sustainable philosophy of green dentistry is in line with the increasing recognition of the relationship between ecological well-being and oral health.

Reducing The Environmental Effects Of Dental Care

Dental professionals can help to reduce the environmental impact of their work by taking a multifaceted approach that addresses different aspects of the dental practice. One important aspect of this approach is waste management, where materials are reduced, reused, and recycled whenever possible. Another important aspect is the responsible sourcing of dental materials, such as recyclable or biodegradable packaging, which helps to create a more sustainable workflow. Finally, energy consumption is a crucial factor that encourages the use of energy-efficient technologies and practices in dental clinics.

As the dental profession develops, incorporating these principles becomes essential for practitioners committed to a holistic approach to patient care and environmental stewardship. These three interrelated concepts together form a holistic framework for sustainable dentistry, acknowledging the complex relationship between oral health and environmental well-being.

CHAPTER 9
HOLISTIC SOLUTIONS FOR FREQUENTLY ASKED DENTAL QUESTIONS

Integrating alternative therapies like oil pulling, herbal remedies, and topical applications of substances like propolis, holistic dentistry aims to address cavities in a way that supports the body's overall well-being. Holistic practitioners emphasize preventive measures, including dietary changes, proper oral hygiene, and nutritional supplements. One aspect of holistic dentistry focuses on natural remedies for cavities, acknowledging that the conventional approach of drilling and filling may not be the only solution.

Another area where holistic dentistry deviates from conventional medicine is in treating gum disease, a common dental condition. Holistic treatments for gum disease emphasize a multimodal approach that includes treating the disease's underlying causes as well as its symptoms; these may include dietary adjustments, lifestyle adjustments, and natural remedies like essential oils, herbal mouthwashes, and colloidal silver, which are known to have antimicrobial properties. By taking into account the connection between oral and general health, holistic dentistry aims to promote a sustainable and balanced solution to gum disease.

To treat tooth sensitivity, which is a common complaint among people, holistic dentists look into the underlying factors that may be causing the condition. They acknowledge that sensitivity can originate from different sources, such as exposed dentin, enamel erosion, or underlying health issues. While traditional dentistry approaches often involve desensitizing toothpaste or fluoride treatments, holistic dentistry goes beyond surface-level solutions and looks for and treats the root causes, which may include nutritional deficiencies, systemic inflammation, or improper oral care practices.

The adoption of a holistic approach to common dental problems represents a paradigm shift in dentistry, moving away from isolated treatments and toward a more integrative and patient-centered approach. This viewpoint acknowledges the complex relationship between oral health and an individual's overall well-being, recognizing that the mouth is a gateway to the body. Holistic dentistry embraces natural remedies, customized treatment plans, and a focus on prevention to provide more long-lasting solutions to common dental problems, ultimately contributing to the individual's holistic health.

Comprehensive Methods For Preventive Dental Care

Holistic dentistry encourages a shift from reactive treatments to preventive strategies, aiming to identify and address potential issues before they escalate. This approach includes patient education on proper oral hygiene practices, personalized dietary recommendations, and lifestyle modifications to reduce risk factors associated with common dental problems.

Preventive dentistry is a cornerstone of holistic approaches to oral health, emphasizing the importance of proactive measures to maintain optimal well-being.

Preventive care in holistic dentistry goes beyond standard procedures like cleanings and exams; instead, it focuses on enabling people to take charge of their oral health via awareness and deliberate decision-making. Examples of such interventions include teaching patients about the relationship between nutrition and oral health, offering advice on minimizing exposure to environmental toxins that can negatively impact oral health, and incorporating oil pulling as a means of preserving a healthy oral microbiome.

Moreover, holistic preventive dentistry acknowledges the relationship between systemic health and oral health. Treating underlying problems like immune system imbalances, chronic inflammation, and nutritional deficiencies, holistic practitioners work to create a healthy environment that lowers the risk of dental problems. This all-encompassing approach to preventive dentistry is consistent with the holistic philosophy of treating the whole person instead of isolated symptoms.

Recognizing the impact of stress on oral health, holistic dentists may include relaxation techniques, meditation, or other stress management strategies in their recommendations. By addressing both the physical and emotional aspects of oral health, holistic dentistry aims to provide a more holistic and sustainable approach to preventive care. Holistic dentistry also emphasizes the role of mindfulness and stress reduction in preventive oral care.

holistic approaches to preventive dentistry emphasize proactive measures to maintain optimal oral health rather than the traditional focus on treating existing conditions.

Holistic dentistry integrates lifestyle modifications, education, and an emphasis on overall well-being to empower people to take charge of their oral health and contribute to their overall holistic well-being.

Comprehensive Methods For Cosmetic Dentistry

Holistic cosmetic dentistry emphasizes procedures that not only improve appearance but also positively impact the patient's overall well-being, going beyond the traditional focus on aesthetics to take into account the individual's overall well-being. Holistic cosmetic dentistry acknowledges the connection between oral health and mental and emotional health.

The use of biocompatible materials in restorative and cosmetic procedures is one facet of holistic cosmetic dentistry. Holistic dentists prioritize materials that are biocompatible to the body, minimizing the risk of adverse reactions or sensitivities. Porcelain veneers, composite resins, and other materials that are in line with the body's natural composition are examples of materials that are compatible with the body. By emphasizing biocompatibility, holistic cosmetic dentistry seeks to promote long-term oral health and minimize the possibility of systemic problems relating to dental materials.

Furthermore, conservative methods that preserve as much of the natural tooth structure as possible are sought after by holistic practitioners of cosmetic dentistry. This approach is consistent with the holistic philosophy of honoring the body's inherent healing capacity and minimizing needless interventions. Holistic practitioners also place a strong emphasis on minimally invasive procedures.

Holistic cosmetic dentistry considers the psychological and emotional effects of dental procedures in addition to the physical ones. Its practitioners take into account the patient's overall well-being, which includes their mental health and self-esteem. Open communication, mindfulness practices, and relaxation techniques are all incorporated into the cosmetic dentistry process to guarantee that the patient has a positive and holistic experience.

holistic approaches to cosmetic dentistry place equal weight on the patient's overall health and aesthetic results. They do this by selecting biocompatible materials, utilizing minimally invasive procedures, and attending to the emotional effects of cosmetic procedures. In short, holistic cosmetic dentistry aims to improve the patient's overall health and appearance while also reflecting a patient-centered philosophy that is consistent with the tenets of holistic dentistry.

CHAPTER 10
HOLISTIC DENTISTRY'S FUTURE
New Developments In Holistic Dental Practice:

Holistic dentistry is experiencing a paradigm shift as emerging trends reshape the landscape of oral health care. One prominent trend is the integration of alternative and complementary therapies with conventional dental practices.

This approach acknowledges the interconnectedness of oral health with overall well-being, emphasizing the importance of addressing root causes rather than just symptoms. The use of biocompatible materials in dental procedures is gaining traction, focusing on materials that are harmonious with the body and minimizing the risk of adverse reactions. Additionally, the incorporation of advanced technologies, such as laser dentistry and digital diagnostics, allows for more precise and minimally invasive treatments, aligning with holistic principles that prioritize patient comfort and systemic health. As holistic dentistry evolves, the emphasis on preventive measures and patient education is growing, empowering individuals to take an active role in maintaining their oral health.

Innovation And Research In Oral Health

The future of holistic dentistry is intricately tied to ongoing research and innovation in oral health. Researchers are delving into the intricate connections between oral health and systemic conditions, uncovering links between periodontal disease and conditions such as cardiovascular disease, diabetes, and respiratory disorders.

This deeper understanding underscores the importance of a holistic approach that considers the entire body in dental care. Innovations in diagnostic tools, such as saliva-based biomarkers and genetic testing, enable personalized and targeted treatments, contributing to a more holistic and patient-centric approach.

The integration of regenerative therapies, such as stem cell applications in periodontal treatments, showcases the potential for transformative breakthroughs in restoring oral health. As research continues to unveil the complexities of oral-systemic connections, holistic dentistry is poised to play a pivotal role in shaping the future of comprehensive and integrative oral health care.

A Comprehensive Perspective On Dentistry's Future:

The evolution towards a more holistic approach in dentistry's future is characterized by a fundamental shift in the way oral health is perceived and managed. Holistic dentistry goes beyond treating symptoms and aims to identify and address the underlying causes of oral health issues.

This involves considering the physical, emotional, and environmental factors that impact an individual's well-being. The future of holistic dentistry embraces a collaborative and interdisciplinary approach, fostering partnerships between dentists, physicians, nutritionists, and other healthcare professionals.

Integrating mindfulness and stress reduction techniques into dental care practices acknowledges the intricate mind-body connection and promotes overall health.

Additionally, community-based preventive programs and outreach initiatives become integral components, emphasizing education and access to holistic dental care for diverse populations.

As the profession evolves, ethical considerations surrounding sustainability, waste reduction, and eco-friendly practices become paramount, aligning with the holistic philosophy that values the health of individuals and the planet.

CONCLUSION

Summary Of The Main Holistic Ideas

Key concepts that redefine the way oral health care is provided include: the recognition of the connection between oral health and overall well-being; prevention as a cornerstone, which encourages proactive measures to maintain optimal oral health and prevent systemic health issues; patient-centered care, which focuses on customized treatment plans that take into account each patient's unique needs and circumstances; biocompatibility and the use of minimally invasive techniques as a means of demonstrating a commitment to holistic principles and guaranteeing that dental interventions are in harmony with the body's natural processes; and the integration of advanced technologies, alternative therapies, and continuing education

Promoting A Comprehensive Strategy For Dental Health

Encouraging a holistic approach to oral health involves a multifaceted strategy that encompasses education, collaboration, and advocacy.

Public awareness campaigns play a crucial role in disseminating information about the interconnected nature of oral and systemic health, fostering a proactive attitude toward preventive care. Collaboration between dental professionals and other healthcare practitioners is essential, promoting an integrated and comprehensive approach to patient care.

Educational programs in dental schools should incorporate holistic principles into their curricula, preparing the next generation of dentists to embrace a broader perspective on oral health.

Furthermore, advocacy for policy changes that support holistic dentistry practices, including insurance coverage for complementary therapies and recognition of the importance of preventive measures, is vital. By collectively embracing and promoting a holistic approach to oral health, individuals, healthcare professionals, and policymakers can contribute to a future where holistic dentistry becomes the standard of care, prioritizing the well-being of individuals and communities alike.

www.ingramcontent.com/pod-product-compliance
Lightning Source LLC
Chambersburg PA
CBHW071102260726
48661CB00006B/2418